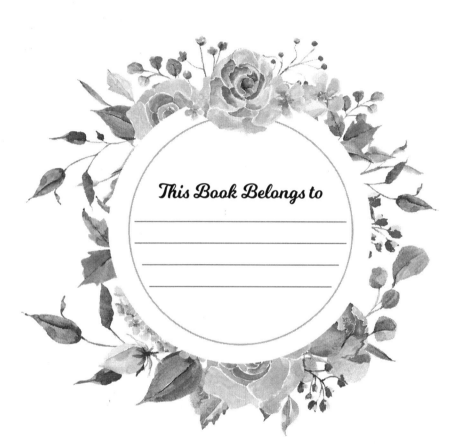

This Book Belongs to

_____
_____
_____
_____

Patient Index

Date	Patient	Page

Patient Index

Date	Patient	Page

Patient Index

Date	Patient	Page

Patient Index

Date	Patient	Page

Patient Name :

Scheduled / PRN :   Mileage :

Time Visit Began :   Time Visit Ended :

Temp :

B / P :

Resp Rate :

Heart Rate :

SO2 :

O2 LPM :

Pain :

Last BM :

Weight :

Left MAC :

Right MAC :

Other :

Current Patient Pain

Oriented To

Family / Facility Updated

Next Visit Date

Patient Name :

Scheduled / PRN :   **Mileage :**

Time Visit Began :   **Time Visit Ended :**

Temp :

B / P :

Resp Rate :

Heart Rate :

SO2 :

O2 LPM :

Pain :

Last BM :

Weight :

Left MAC :

Right MAC :

Other :

Current Patient Pain

Oriented To

Family / Facility Updated

Next Visit Date

Patient Name :

Scheduled / PRN :   Mileage :

Time Visit Began :   Time Visit Ended :

Temp :

B / P :

Resp Rate :

Heart Rate :

SO2 :

O2 LPM :

Pain :

Last BM :

Weight :

Left MAC :

Right MAC :

Other :

Current Patient Pain

Oriented To

Family / Facility Updated

Next Visit Date

Patient Name :

Scheduled / PRN :   Mileage :

Time Visit Began :   Time Visit Ended :

Temp :

B / P :

Resp Rate :

Heart Rate :

SO2 :

O2 LPM :

Pain :

Last BM :

Weight :

Left MAC :

Right MAC :

Other :

Current Patient Pain

Oriented To

Family / Facility Updated

Next Visit Date

Patient Name :

Scheduled / PRN :   Mileage :

Time Visit Began :   Time Visit Ended :

Temp :   **Current Patient Pain**

B / P :

Resp Rate :

Heart Rate :

SO2 :

O2 LPM :   **Oriented To**

Pain :

Last BM :

Weight :

Left MAC :

Right MAC :   **Family / Facility Updated**

Other :

                                     Next Visit Date

Patient Name :

Scheduled / PRN :   **Mileage :**

Time Visit Began :   **Time Visit Ended :**

Temp :

B / P :

Resp Rate :

Heart Rate :

SO2 :

O2 LPM :

Pain :

Last BM :

Weight :

Left MAC :

Right MAC :

Current Patient Pain

Oriented To

Family / Facility Updated

Other :

Next Visit Date

Patient Name :

Scheduled / PRN :   Mileage :

Time Visit Began :   Time Visit Ended :

Temp :   Current Patient Pain

B / P :

Resp Rate :

Heart Rate :

SO2 :

O2 LPM :   Oriented To

Pain :

Last BM :

Weight :

Left MAC :

Right MAC :   Family / Facility Updated

Other :

                                               Next Visit Date

Patient Name :

Scheduled / PRN :　　　　　　Mileage :

Time Visit Began :　　　　　　Time Visit Ended :

Temp :　　　　　　　　　　　Current Patient Pain

B / P :

Resp Rate :

Heart Rate :

SO2 :

O2 LPM :　　　　　　　　　　Oriented To

Pain :

Last BM :

Weight :

Left MAC :

Right MAC :　　　　　　　　Family / Facility Updated

Other :

Next Visit Date

Patient Name :

Scheduled / PRN :   Mileage :

Time Visit Began :   Time Visit Ended :

Temp :   Current Patient Pain

B / P :

Resp Rate :

Heart Rate :

SO2 :

O2 LPM :   Oriented To

Pain :

Last BM :

Weight :

Left MAC :

Right MAC :   Family / Facility Updated

Other :

                                     Next Visit Date

Patient Name :

Scheduled / PRN :　　　　Mileage :

Time Visit Began :　　　　Time Visit Ended :

Temp :

B / P :

Resp Rate :

Heart Rate :

SO2 :

O2 LPM :

Pain :

Last BM :

Weight :

Left MAC :

Right MAC :

Other :

Current Patient Pain

Oriented To

Family / Facility Updated

Next Visit Date

Patient Name :

Scheduled / PRN :　　　Mileage :

Time Visit Began :　　　Time Visit Ended :

Temp :

B / P :

Resp Rate :

Heart Rate :

SO2 :

O2 LPM :

Pain :

Last BM :

Weight :

Left MAC :

Right MAC :

Other :

Current Patient Pain

Oriented To

Family / Facility Updated

Next Visit Date

Patient Name :

Scheduled / PRN :   Mileage :

Time Visit Began :   Time Visit Ended :

Temp :

B / P :

Resp Rate :

Heart Rate :

SO2 :

O2 LPM :

Pain :

Last BM :

Weight :

Left MAC :

Right MAC :

Other :

Current Patient Pain

Oriented To

Family / Facility Updated

Next Visit Date

Patient Name :

Scheduled / PRN :   Mileage :

Time Visit Began :   Time Visit Ended :

Temp :

B / P :

Resp Rate :

Heart Rate :

SO2 :

O2 LPM :

Pain :

Last BM :

Weight :

Left MAC :

Right MAC :

Other :

Current Patient Pain

Oriented To

Family / Facility Updated

Next Visit Date

Patient Name :

Scheduled / PRN :   Mileage :

Time Visit Began :   Time Visit Ended :

Temp :   **Current Patient Pain**

B / P :

Resp Rate :

Heart Rate :

SO2 :

O2 LPM :   **Oriented To**

Pain :

Last BM :

Weight :

Left MAC :

Right MAC :   **Family / Facility Updated**

Other :

                                      Next Visit Date

(M) T (W) T (F) S (S

M T W T F S S

Date : _____

Patient Name :

Scheduled / PRN :   Mileage :

Time Visit Began :   Time Visit Ended :

Temp :   Current Patient Pain

B / P :

Resp Rate :

Heart Rate :

SO2 :

O2 LPM :   Oriented To

Pain :

Last BM :

Weight :

Left MAC :

Right MAC :   Family / Facility Updated

Other :

Next Visit Date

Patient Name :

Scheduled / PRN :   Mileage :

Time Visit Began :   Time Visit Ended :

Temp :   Current Patient Pain

B / P :

Resp Rate :

Heart Rate :

SO2 :

O2 LPM :   Oriented To

Pain :

Last BM :

Weight :

Left MAC :

Right MAC :   Family / Facility Updated

Other :

                                     Next Visit Date

Patient Name :

Scheduled / PRN :   Mileage :

Time Visit Began :   Time Visit Ended :

Temp :

B / P :

Resp Rate :

Heart Rate :

SO2 :

O2 LPM :

Pain :

Last BM :

Weight :

Left MAC :

Right MAC :

Other :

Current Patient Pain

Oriented To

Family / Facility Updated

Next Visit Date

Patient Name :

Scheduled / PRN :   Mileage :

Time Visit Began :   Time Visit Ended :

Temp :

B / P :

Resp Rate :

Heart Rate :

SO2 :

O2 LPM :

Pain :

Last BM :

Weight :

Left MAC :

Right MAC :

Other :

Current Patient Pain

Oriented To

Family / Facility Updated

Next Visit Date

Patient Name :

Scheduled / PRN :

Time Visit Began :

Mileage :

Time Visit Ended :

Temp :

B / P :

Resp Rate :

Heart Rate :

SO2 :

O2 LPM :

Pain :

Last BM :

Weight :

Left MAC :

Right MAC :

Other :

Current Patient Pain

Oriented To

Family / Facility Updated

Next Visit Date

Patient Name :

Scheduled / PRN :   Mileage :

Time Visit Began :   Time Visit Ended :

Temp :

B / P :

Resp Rate :

Heart Rate :

SO2 :

O2 LPM :

Pain :

Last BM :

Weight :

Left MAC :

Right MAC :

Other :

Current Patient Pain

Oriented To

Family / Facility Updated

Next Visit Date

Patient Name :

Scheduled / PRN :

Mileage :

Time Visit Began :

Time Visit Ended :

Temp :

B / P :

Resp Rate :

Heart Rate :

SO2 :

O2 LPM :

Pain :

Last BM :

Weight :

Left MAC :

Right MAC :

Current Patient Pain

Oriented To

Family / Facility Updated

Next Visit Date

Other :

Patient Name :

Scheduled / PRN :   Mileage :

Time Visit Began :   Time Visit Ended :

Temp :   Current Patient Pain

B / P :

Resp Rate :

Heart Rate :

SO2 :

O2 LPM :   Oriented To

Pain :

Last BM :

Weight :

Left MAC :

Right MAC :   Family / Facility Updated

Other :

                                     Next Visit Date

📅 Date : . . . .

Patient Name :

Scheduled / PRN :   Mileage :

Time Visit Began :   Time Visit Ended :

Temp :

B / P :

Resp Rate :

Heart Rate :

SO2 :

O2 LPM :

Pain :

Last BM :

Weight :

Left MAC :

Right MAC :

Current Patient Pain

Oriented To

Family / Facility Updated

Other :

Next Visit Date

Patient Name :

Scheduled / PRN :   Mileage :

Time Visit Began :   Time Visit Ended :

Temp :

B / P :

Resp Rate :

Heart Rate :

SO2 :

O2 LPM :

Pain :

Last BM :

Weight :

Left MAC :

Right MAC :

Other :

Current Patient Pain

Oriented To

Family / Facility Updated

Next Visit Date

Patient Name :

Scheduled / PRN :   Mileage :

Time Visit Began :   Time Visit Ended :

Temp :

B / P :

Resp Rate :

Heart Rate :

SO2 :

O2 LPM :

Pain :

Last BM :

Weight :

Left MAC :

Right MAC :

Other :

Current Patient Pain

Oriented To

Family / Facility Updated

Next Visit Date

Patient Name :

Scheduled / PRN :   Mileage :

Time Visit Began :   Time Visit Ended :

Temp :   **Current Patient Pain**

B / P :

Resp Rate :

Heart Rate :

SO2 :

O2 LPM :   **Oriented To**

Pain :

Last BM :

Weight :

Left MAC :

Right MAC :   **Family / Facility Updated**

Other :

                                     Next Visit Date

Patient Name :

Scheduled / PRN :   Mileage :

Time Visit Began :   Time Visit Ended :

Temp :

B / P :

Resp Rate :

Heart Rate :

SO2 :

O2 LPM :

Pain :

Last BM :

Weight :

Left MAC :

Right MAC :

Other :

Current Patient Pain

Oriented To

Family / Facility Updated

Next Visit Date

Patient Name :

Scheduled / PRN :   Mileage :

Time Visit Began :   Time Visit Ended :

Temp :   Current Patient Pain

B / P :

Resp Rate :

Heart Rate :

SO2 :

O2 LPM :   Oriented To

Pain :

Last BM :

Weight :

Left MAC :

Right MAC :   Family / Facility Updated

Other :

                               Next Visit Date

Patient Name :

Scheduled / PRN :   Mileage :

Time Visit Began :   Time Visit Ended :

Temp :

B / P :

Resp Rate :

Heart Rate :

SO2 :

O2 LPM :

Pain :

Last BM :

Weight :

Left MAC :

Right MAC :

Other :

Current Patient Pain

Oriented To

Family / Facility Updated

Next Visit Date

Patient Name :

Scheduled / PRN :　　　Mileage :

Time Visit Began :　　　Time Visit Ended :

Temp :

B / P :

Resp Rate :

Heart Rate :

SO2 :

O2 LPM :

Pain :

Last BM :

Weight :

Left MAC :

Right MAC :

Other :

Current Patient Pain

Oriented To

Family / Facility Updated

Next Visit Date

Patient Name :

Scheduled / PRN : Mileage :

Time Visit Began : Time Visit Ended :

Temp :

B / P :

Resp Rate :

Heart Rate :

SO2 :

O2 LPM :

Pain :

Last BM :

Weight :

Left MAC :

Right MAC :

Other :

Current Patient Pain

Oriented To

Family / Facility Updated

Next Visit Date

Patient Name :

Scheduled / PRN :

Mileage :

Time Visit Began :

Time Visit Ended :

Temp :

B / P :

Resp Rate :

Heart Rate :

SO2 :

O2 LPM :

Pain :

Last BM :

Weight :

Left MAC :

Right MAC :

Other :

Current Patient Pain

Oriented To

Family / Facility Updated

Next Visit Date

Patient Name :

Scheduled / PRN :

Mileage :

Time Visit Began :

Time Visit Ended :

Temp :

B / P :

Resp Rate :

Heart Rate :

SO2 :

O2 LPM :

Pain :

Last BM :

Weight :

Left MAC :

Right MAC :

Other :

Current Patient Pain

Oriented To

Family / Facility Updated

Next Visit Date

Patient Name :

Scheduled / PRN :   Mileage :

Time Visit Began :   Time Visit Ended :

Temp :   Current Patient Pain

B / P :

Resp Rate :

Heart Rate :

SO2 :

O2 LPM :   Oriented To

Pain :

Last BM :

Weight :

Left MAC :

Right MAC :   Family / Facility Updated

Other :

Next Visit Date

Patient Name :

Scheduled / PRN :   Mileage :

Time Visit Began :   Time Visit Ended :

Temp :

B / P :

Resp Rate :

Heart Rate :

SO2 :

O2 LPM :

Pain :

Last BM :

Weight :

Left MAC :

Right MAC :

Other :

Current Patient Pain

Oriented To

Family / Facility Updated

Next Visit Date

Patient Name :

Scheduled / PRN :   Mileage :

Time Visit Began :   Time Visit Ended :

Temp :   Current Patient Pain

B / P :

Resp Rate :

Heart Rate :

SO2 :

O2 LPM :   Oriented To

Pain :

Last BM :

Weight :

Left MAC :

Right MAC :   Family / Facility Updated

Other :

                                           Next Visit Date

Patient Name :

Scheduled / PRN :   Mileage :

Time Visit Began :   Time Visit Ended :

Temp :

B / P :

Resp Rate :

Heart Rate :

SO2 :

O2 LPM :

Pain :

Last BM :

Weight :

Left MAC :

Right MAC :

Other :

Current Patient Pain

Oriented To

Family / Facility Updated

Next Visit Date

Patient Name :

Scheduled / PRN :   Mileage :

Time Visit Began :   Time Visit Ended :

Temp :

B / P :

Resp Rate :

Heart Rate :

SO2 :

O2 LPM :

Pain :

Last BM :

Weight :

Left MAC :

Right MAC :

Other :

Current Patient Pain

Oriented To

Family / Facility Updated

Next Visit Date

Patient Name :

Scheduled / PRN :   Mileage :

Time Visit Began :   Time Visit Ended :

Temp :   Current Patient Pain

B / P :

Resp Rate :

Heart Rate :

SO2 :

O2 LPM :   Oriented To

Pain :

Last BM :

Weight :

Left MAC :

Right MAC :   Family / Facility Updated

Other :

                                     Next Visit Date

Patient Name :

Scheduled / PRN :   Mileage :

Time Visit Began :   Time Visit Ended :

Temp :

B / P :

Resp Rate :

Heart Rate :

SO2 :

O2 LPM :

Pain :

Last BM :

Weight :

Left MAC :

Right MAC :

Other :

Current Patient Pain

Oriented To

Family / Facility Updated

Next Visit Date

Patient Name :

Scheduled / PRN :   Mileage :

Time Visit Began :   Time Visit Ended :

Temp :

B / P :

Resp Rate :

Heart Rate :

SO2 :

O2 LPM :

Pain :

Last BM :

Weight :

Left MAC :

Right MAC :

Other :

Current Patient Pain

Oriented To

Family / Facility Updated

Next Visit Date

Patient Name :

Scheduled / PRN :   **Mileage :**

Time Visit Began :   **Time Visit Ended :**

Temp :

B / P :

Resp Rate :

Heart Rate :

SO2 :

O2 LPM :

Pain :

Last BM :

Weight :

Left MAC :

Right MAC :

Other :

Current Patient Pain

Oriented To

Family / Facility Updated

Next Visit Date

Patient Name :

Scheduled / PRN :   Mileage :

Time Visit Began :   Time Visit Ended :

Temp :   Current Patient Pain

B / P :

Resp Rate :

Heart Rate :

SO2 :

O2 LPM :   Oriented To

Pain :

Last BM :

Weight :

Left MAC :

Right MAC :   Family / Facility Updated

Other :

                                       Next Visit Date

Patient Name :

Scheduled / PRN :   Mileage :

Time Visit Began :   Time Visit Ended :

Temp :   **Current Patient Pain**

B / P :

Resp Rate :

Heart Rate :

SO2 :

O2 LPM :   **Oriented To**

Pain :

Last BM :

Weight :

Left MAC :

Right MAC :   **Family / Facility Updated**

Other :

                                     Next Visit Date

Patient Name :

Scheduled / PRN :   Mileage :

Time Visit Began :   Time Visit Ended :

Temp :

B / P :

Resp Rate :

Heart Rate :

SO2 :

O2 LPM :

Pain :

Last BM :

Weight :

Left MAC :

Right MAC :

Other :

Current Patient Pain

Oriented To

Family / Facility Updated

Next Visit Date

Patient Name :

Scheduled / PRN :   Mileage :

Time Visit Began :   Time Visit Ended :

Temp :   Current Patient Pain

B / P :

Resp Rate :

Heart Rate :

SO2 :

O2 LPM :   Oriented To

Pain :

Last BM :

Weight :

Left MAC :

Right MAC :   Family / Facility Updated

Other :

Next Visit Date

Patient Name :

Scheduled / PRN :   Mileage :

Time Visit Began :   Time Visit Ended :

Temp :

B / P :

Resp Rate :

Heart Rate :

SO2 :

O2 LPM :

Pain :

Last BM :

Weight :

Left MAC :

Right MAC :

Other :

Current Patient Pain

Oriented To

Family / Facility Updated

Next Visit Date

Patient Name :

Scheduled / PRN :   Mileage :

Time Visit Began :   Time Visit Ended :

Temp :

B / P :

Resp Rate :

Heart Rate :

SO2 :

O2 LPM :

Pain :

Last BM :

Weight :

Left MAC :

Right MAC :

Other :

Current Patient Pain

Oriented To

Family / Facility Updated

Next Visit Date

Patient Name :

Scheduled / PRN :   Mileage :

Time Visit Began :   Time Visit Ended :

Temp :

B / P :

Resp Rate :

Heart Rate :

SO2 :

O2 LPM :

Pain :

Last BM :

Weight :

Left MAC :

Right MAC :

Other :

Current Patient Pain

Oriented To

Family / Facility Updated

Next Visit Date

Patient Name :

Scheduled / PRN :   Mileage :

Time Visit Began :   Time Visit Ended :

Temp :

B / P :

Resp Rate :

Heart Rate :

SO2 :

O2 LPM :

Pain :

Last BM :

Weight :

Left MAC :

Right MAC :

Other :

Current Patient Pain

Oriented To

Family / Facility Updated

Next Visit Date

Patient Name :

Scheduled / PRN :   Mileage :

Time Visit Began :   Time Visit Ended :

Temp :   Current Patient Pain

B / P :

Resp Rate :

Heart Rate :

SO2 :

O2 LPM :   Oriented To

Pain :

Last BM :

Weight :

Left MAC :

Right MAC :   Family / Facility Updated

Other :

                                 Next Visit Date

Patient Name :

Scheduled / PRN :   Mileage :

Time Visit Began :   Time Visit Ended :

Temp :

B / P :

Resp Rate :

Heart Rate :

SO2 :

O2 LPM :

Pain :

Last BM :

Weight :

Left MAC :

Right MAC :

Other :

Current Patient Pain

Oriented To

Family / Facility Updated

Next Visit Date

Made in the USA
Middletown, DE
08 January 2025

68984526R00062